Cancer Lives
at Our House

Also by Beatrice Hofman Hoek with Melanie Jongsma
Surrender or Fight? One Woman's Victory over Cancer

Cancer Lives at Our House

Help for the Family

Beatrice Hofman Hoek
with Melanie Jongsma

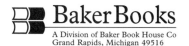
Baker Books
A Division of Baker Book House Co
Grand Rapids, Michigan 49516

©1997 by Beatrice Hofman Hoek

Published by Baker Books
a division of Baker Book House Company
P.O. Box 6287, Grand Rapids, MI 49516-6287

Printed in the United States of America

Library of Congress Cataloging-in-Publication Data

Hoek, Beatrice Hofman, 1941–
    Cancer lives at our house : help for the family /
    Beatrice Hofman Hoek, with Melanie Jongsma.
            p.   cm.
    Includes bibliographical references.
    ISBN 0-8010-5735-3
        1. Cancer—Patients—Family relationships.
    I. Jongsma, Melanie, 1967– . II. Title.
    RC262.H59   1997
    155.9'16—dc20   96-9230

Contents

Foreword

Though cancer is usually described with reference to a single organ (such as "liver cancer"), its victims realize that it is a disease affecting their entire body. There has been a system failure that has caused the body's cells to become enemies of one another. Treatment for cancer affects the entire organism, too, and radiation and chemotherapy make a person feel very unwell—all over.

But this disease not only affects the patient's entire being; it also affects that most delicate and important social organism: the family. The panic that often seizes a cancer patient when the diagnosis is first made, and that soon becomes a confused and abiding dread, is reflected in the patient's spouse, children, and parents. Because we tend to view cancer as terminal and consider survivors as exceptions to a dreadful rule, no one connected with the patient can escape considering the possibility of losing him or her through death.

The impact of this disease on the patient's family is often considered quite secondary, but it is much more than a footnote to the unfolding experience of the cancer sufferer. The fact that cancer invades a home and disrupts its well-being has a direct bearing on the effectiveness of therapies employed and impacts each family member along with the primary sufferer.

Often, cancer survivors will tell you that their experience with the disease was a turning point which led them to a more joy-filled savoring of life's sweetness. And just as often, adolescent children of a parent stricken with cancer will also tell how their mother's or father's cancer became a changing point for them. A family member's cancer is often as traumatic a personal experience as it is for the patient.

In the first book about Bea Hoek's struggle with breast cancer, *Surrender or Fight?*, we learned of the way this illness affected her physically, emotionally, and spiritually. In this sequel, she examines what happened in her family. It is a slender volume, but the openness and candor of her children and her husband make this book exceptionally valuable. We are in Bea's debt for probing, as she has, the feelings of her own family and of other families. Some cancer sufferers remain isolated in their own grief and misery, scarcely suspecting that their dear ones are going through intense experiences as well. Bea has chosen to face this, to examine it and hold it up for all of us to see.

On the pages that follow, we meet Jackie, Jayne, Jon, and husband Jim—four J's who were changed by Bea's experience. And we learn of others who have had to deal with the devastation of this illness in their families. Of special importance are Bea's helpful suggestions to teachers who have family members of cancer patients in their classrooms.

Through it all, there is the calm certainty that God is not surprised by our cancer and that he is in control at every moment while our journey to wellness or toward death gets under way. As we are reminded of Christ's suffering, we remember that when he died, *his* family, too, was affected. His mother watched him die. His Father in heaven hid his face and covered the crucifixion scene with merciful darkness while his Son paid the price for our sin and made ultimate healing possible for all who put their trust in him.

"Praise the LORD, O my soul, and forget not all his benefits—who forgives all your sins and heals all your diseases" (Ps. 103:2–3). As we read Psalm 103, we remember that the Savior heals even our stricken families; they, too, need his healing touch when *Cancer Lives at Our House.*

Joel Nederhood
Retired Director of Ministries
The Back to God Hour/Faith 20

Foreword

Bea Hoek and I share more than a common faith and a European Dutch ancestry. We share a diagnosis of cancer.

Bea was diagnosed with breast cancer in 1983, the same year I was diagnosed with Hodgkin's disease. We are thus both thirteen-year survivors. The images she describes—of cancer initially invading and then living in her household—are strikingly similar to those that occurred in the home that my wife and I had built for our three boys. The memories of words describing the initial diagnosis, the impact of the diagnosis on a twelve-year-old who thought the word *cancer* meant Daddy was going to die, and the strain placed on my wife at a time when we were just beginning a family life together will never be forgotten. I recall vividly (as almost every cancer survivor does) the very first symptoms, the initial doctor visits, the exact type and location of the tests, and the precise events surrounding the treatment and prognosis.

Although cancer induces a type of post-traumatic stress syndrome in everyone, it also includes a post-treatment euphoria. That is what Bea is celebrating in this book. The euphoria of being able to celebrate life abundantly and in God's world. The euphoria of watching our children grow and mature when it was once not clear if we could share those moments at all.

This book is not about cancer. This book is about life—a life to be celebrated, enjoyed, and someday left for an even better life.

Nicholas Vogelzang, M.D.
Professor of Medicine
University of Chicago Hospitals

Preface

When I was first diagnosed with breast cancer in 1983, I was totally overwhelmed. I said to myself, "It would be easier to die than to face multiple surgeries, chemotherapy, radiation, needles, and then uncertainty." I understood why some cancer patients give up. I could even imagine why some commit suicide. The grief and fear are almost inexpressible. The pain doesn't go away. The despair and anxiety are all-consuming.

But later that night I woke up and prayed, "Lord, please don't let me die." I was only forty-two. I wanted to see my children graduate from high school. I wanted to celebrate my twenty-fifth wedding anniversary with the man I loved. I wanted grandchildren and retirement—all the "normal" things.

So I began my war against cancer, my fight for life, which I wrote about in 1995 in *Surrender or*

Fight? One Woman's Victory over Cancer. That fight goes on today and probably will for the rest of my life. What I have become increasingly aware of, however, is that my cancer presented a battle not only for me, but also for my family. And their battle experience was not always the same as mine.

What follows is a journal of my family's response to my cancer, as well as insights from friends and acquaintances who have been involved at some level in a struggle with cancer. It is my prayer that others who face cancer and its emotional fallout will find they are not alone and will avail themselves of the peace that comes through total surrender to God's loving care.

Beatrice Hofman Hoek

1

What's All the Fighting For?

My daughter Jackie was eleven years old when I was diagnosed with cancer, perhaps too young to understand much of what was going on. Before my diagnosis she had been a sixth-grade sports fanatic. She tried out for every team she could think of, and made most of them. When she wasn't at a tryout or a practice or a game of some sort, she was at a friend's birthday party or a sleep over. She was also learning to balance her active social life with the responsibility of a paper route. Jackie was a normal kid, completely unaware of how her life would be changed by my illness.

I'm not sure how Jackie reacted to the news of my diagnosis—I was so wrapped up in the over-whelming unbelievability of it all that I couldn't think of how my family was responding. It's not that I was *unaware* of my family—in fact, they were the primary motivation behind my struggle to live. But during the early stages of my battle I was most often consumed with my own emotions, and I tended to assume that my family was reacting to everything the same way I was. In Jackie's case that wasn't always true. She remembers:

> Sixth grade was one of the turning points in my life. However, I didn't realize that until later. This was the year that my mom found a lump in her breast.
>
> I can remember the exact day my parents told me about this. Mom was sitting on her bed, and Dad was sitting right next to her. Dad said to me, "Mom has a lump in her breast." I did not really know what was going on at the time, but all of a sudden things became very hectic around the house, and I could feel the stress and tension in the air. Someone finally sat me down and told me Mom had breast cancer.
>
> Mom would go to the hospital all the time, and sometimes she would be gone for days. I remember spending a lot of time staying with friends or relatives. I remember the house being full of flowers, food, books, and visitors. I remember Mom being ex-hausted and depressed. And I remember people always asking me, "How's your mother?"

I started learning new words like *chemotherapy* and *radiation,* which I didn't understand. All I knew was that Mom was getting very skinny, and she seemed sick all the time.

This was a very hectic time in my life. I was miserable. At one point I finally started to realize that I didn't know if Mom was going to be alive to see me graduate from eighth grade.

Jackie, I think, was more angry than our other children at cancer's invasion of our home and domination of our lives. She resented the threat that it posed to her mother, but she also resented the fact that defeating cancer would take up most of our time. There wasn't any "normal" anymore. A life of trips to the local pool and inviting friends overnight had been replaced with a life of "Shhh, Mom's resting." Before my cancer, Jackie could be the center of my attention. Now I had to be the center of hers—and everyone else's. Cancer had moved in and taken over, and she could not forgive it.

Even now, thirteen years later, cancer lives at our house. I spend a lot of my time counseling other cancer patients over the phone, writing and speaking about my experience, reading the latest books on the subject, going to the hospital for regular checkups and tests. And Jackie still carries around some of the resentment she has felt from the start.

Of course, I had been largely oblivious of what Jackie was feeling, and when she finally began expressing it, I was taken aback. I had fought so hard to survive for my family, for my children—and *this* was how they responded? To be honest, it seemed to me that my daughter was being selfish. I didn't understand the depth of her pain. I didn't realize that she had been a victim of cancer's attack as well. To make matters worse, I mistook her resentment of the cancer as resentment of *me,* and I was hurt. Of course, the cancer and I were so closely intertwined that Jackie may not always have been sure at which she was directing her emotions, and that only served to make the whole issue harder to talk about.

My daughter's anger and resentment were not all-consuming, however. She did what she could to respond in encouraging and positive ways. She prayed earnestly and faithfully. She offered to help me change the dressings on my radiation burns. And she wrote out special Bible verses for me when she knew another hurdle lay ahead.

The LORD is a refuge for the oppressed, a stronghold in times of trouble. Psalm 9:9
God bless, Mom! Just trust in God. He'll carry you through.

Love ya!
Jackie

Jackie and I are still sorting through our feelings. Our relationship is still sometimes tense and strained. We have both hurt and been hurt. But in talking with other cancer survivors and their families, we have found that we are not alone. Jackie's feelings are perfectly normal and understandable. If I am wise, I will accept them—and help her to accept them too.

2

The Invisible Victims

Jackie's unexpected response to the whole cancer struggle opened my eyes to the farther-reaching effects of diagnosis and treatment. The battle was overwhelming and traumatic for me, but it seemed to be essentially *my* battle. I was the most visible victim, so I received the most support: prayers, letters, hugs, visitors, favors, and other expressions of concern. As I wrote in *Surrender or Fight?*, "In one sense, I was alone with my cancer. No one else in the world could understand what I was going through. But in another sense, we Christians are never alone, because we are part of the body of Christ. Al-

23

though our functions and situations are unique, we are all intricately bound together by his love and ultimate purpose. The love I felt from the family of God was a source of strength throughout my struggle."

Immersed in my own thoughts, decisions, medical regimen, and alternating feelings, I was unaware of the depth of the struggle my family was going through. And *they* didn't receive nearly as much support as I did from our wider circle of friends. My family became the "invisible victims."

In fact, in some ways a cancer patient's family has a *more* difficult struggle. The patient is "allowed" to express troublesome feelings like fear, despair, and grief, whereas the family feels the heavy burden of keeping a positive attitude, being "brave" and encouraging. The patient's battle is more clearly focused on the cancer itself. But family members may find themselves changing targets and tactics—from being supportive, to trying to motivate the patient, to accepting difficult decisions—all while keeping their own feelings carefully concealed.

If you know someone who is battling cancer, be aware of the invisible victims as well. Pray for the whole family. Be sensitive to their special emotional needs, but realize that they may not want to talk about cancer all the time. Even when you send a card to the patient, remember the family members too.

Reach out especially to the children. You may be able to give them a break from the constant presence of cancer in their home by inviting them to a movie or a day at the zoo. You might help out in practical ways by offering to pick them up from school, bring them to a doctor's or haircut appointment, or take them shopping for school supplies. Let them know that they are still special by remembering to send a card on their birthdays. In short, do whatever you can to recognize and affirm their identity outside of the cancer experience.

Remember that it can be difficult for family members to ask for help. Don't just say, "If there's anything I can do . . ." Take the first step and volunteer to do something specific.

And be patient. Be aware that the emotional battles of the invisible victims may show up in unexpected and uncomfortable ways. Children may have temper tantrums or withdraw into sullenness. Spouses may burst into tears at odd times. Don't be afraid of these expressions, and try not to exacerbate the problem by avoiding the family. Do what you can to let the sufferer know that his or her feelings are valid, even though they may be confusing.

> Blest be the tie that binds
> Our hearts in Christian love!
> The fellowship of kindred minds
> Is like to that above.

Cancer Lives at Our House

Before our Father's throne
  We pour our ardent prayers;
Our fears, our hopes, our aims are one,
  Our comforts and our cares.

We share our mutual woes,
  Our mutual burdens bear;
And often for each other flows
  The sympathizing tear.
John Fawcett

All suffering is difficult to bear, but silence makes the suffering worse. The apostle Paul instructs us to "Carry each other's burdens" (Gal. 6:2). In so doing, let us not forget the burdens of cancer's invisible victims.

3

Dealing with Denial

Our daughter Jayne was a high school sophomore when we received the news about my cancer. She was shocked and scared by the diagnosis, of course, but she doesn't remember much about any other feelings she had. "I wish I could remember more about how I felt," she says today, "but I was sort of numb and in a daze about the seriousness of it all. It was a very strange feeling. My days at school seemed pretty normal, and it didn't seem to affect me much. I did not think about the situation. It was kind of just there. It wasn't like I wasn't concerned—because I was—but I just did not want to face it. I would go on each day, and everything

I was involved in at school put my mind off the situation at home. But yet, deep down, I knew that this could change my life." Jayne was in denial.

In some ways the seriousness of my illness was easy for her to deny—I didn't *look* like the typical cancer patient. Jayne had heard, for example, that the chemotherapy and radiation could make me very sick and might make my hair fall out. Those things didn't happen to me. I was often exhausted and nauseous, and I'm sure I didn't look fit and healthy all the time, but I was still recognizable. This may have made it easier for my daughter to believe that my death from this disease was not a real possibility. She says, "For the most part, things seemed almost normal, and that was just the way I liked it. I wanted to go on with life as if this was a little bit of a distraction and then over time things would be the same again. I kept telling myself, 'She'll get better' and 'This isn't so bad.' I don't think I allowed myself to think about cancer and death very deeply, because it would have been too painful."

Jayne's denial was actually a blessing to me in many ways, because it put her in a good position to minister. She cut back on some of her activities at school to spend time with me—reading the Bible or praying or just talking. I appreciated her optimism and the way she tried to cling to normalcy, even though I was concerned about her seeming inability to accept the possibility of my death.

Mon. Feb. 6, 1984
Mom,
    Just wanted to let you know I'll be thinking
of you today—just like every other day! I'm so
glad you're doing so well. I pray for you all the
time and I'm sure you'll be all better soon.
Thanks for being so positive all the time—it
makes everyone else happy—but don't think you
can't be upset because there's always gonna be
that. Hope everything goes well today and the
rest of the week!
                                    I Love You!
                                    Jayne
P.S. Have a nice day!!

For our family, Jayne's denial did not cause a lot of dramatic emotional fallout—because my struggle with cancer has had a happy ending. Jayne has been able to take all the time she needs to come face to face with her fears. Well, actually, in a sense she never has come face to face with the fears themselves, though now she has at least found the strength to look back at those fears and face the memory of how real they were. In fact, it has only been in the past five years that she's begun to uncover some of her hidden feelings. And even now she says, "I sometimes take it for granted that my mom is healthy and doing well. I'm probably doing a little bit of denying

29

again. I am still afraid of losing my mom. I feel like I couldn't face having her die. When I think back to those events, I get a strange feeling in the pit of my stomach."

I'm not really sure of the best way to deal with denial. As I explained in *Surrender or Fight?*, acceptance of a terminal illness is a thin line between denial and resignation, and walking that thin line is tricky. I knew Jayne was in denial, but I was in no position to minister to her. I was well aware of, and sometimes overwhelmed with, the seriousness of my condition. Yet overwhelming my daughter with it too seemed unnecessary. The most I could do was to give her the freedom to own her own feelings about my cancer and hope that she would.

Perhaps the only way to deal with denial is to let it run its course. After all, at some point all of us will have to face our fears of death and loss of a loved one. Sometimes we are given the time to prepare for it. Sometimes the end comes suddenly, unexpectedly. Either way, life's realities have a way of stripping us of the denials in which we wrap ourselves. So why force early acceptance when acceptance will eventually force itself on us?

God does promise us comfort for every heartbreak we endure. That comfort may seem ineffectual and distant if it's *your* heart that has been recently shattered. But remember, the crux of the matter for Christians is that *this* life's realities are not our ultimate reality. Whatever grief and pain we are forced to accept on this earth will melt into peace one day when we reunite in heaven. And that's a reality no one can deny:

> So will it be with the resurrection of the dead. The body that is sown is perishable, it is raised imperishable; it is sown in dishonor, it is raised in glory; it is sown in weakness, it is raised in power; it is sown a natural body, it is raised a spiritual body.
>
> . . . Listen, I tell you a mystery: We will not all sleep, but we will all be changed—in a flash, in the twinkling of an eye, at the last trumpet. For the trumpet will sound, the dead will be raised imperishable, and we will be changed. . . . [T]hen the saying that is written will come true: "Death has been swallowed up in victory."
>
> 1 Corinthians 15:42–44, 51–54

4

The Green-Eyed Monster

*S*trange as it sounds, it is not at all uncommon for family members—particularly young children—to feel intensely *jealous* of the cancer patient in their midst. I believe jealousy is part of the mix of feelings my youngest child, Jackie, went through during my illness, and I have heard stories from other families about similar reactions.

Marci is one example. When she was only four years old, her five-year-old brother, Brett, was diagnosed with leukemia. Here are some of her memories of that time:

I don't remember registering a big reaction to the news, because at that age I had no concept of death, illness, or intense pain. When Mom said he was very sick, I interpreted that to mean he had the flu or something similar—but with a high fever. I felt sorry for him because it's never fun to be sick.

But as Brett's illness progressed, I started thinking the whole thing was ridiculous. I had been sick before too, but I was always better in a few days. I couldn't understand why this was taking so long—especially when he kept going to the hospital. The hospital was where you went to be made better, but sometimes he'd be worse when he came home. It just didn't make any sense to me.

I was so jealous of him during his treatments. I *wished* I could be so lucky as to have a big disease like he had. Here's why: When he went in for treatments, Mom would go with him and stay glued to his bedside and talk with him and play games with him. When Mom wasn't there, he had twenty-four hours of cartoons on the hospital TV. This seemed like *paradise* to me. Brett got attention from the hospital staff, his doctors, my mom and dad, people from church . . . I, on the other hand, was feeling a bit neglected.

Marci's feelings about her brother's illness are perfectly normal. Kids are by nature egocentric—they simply don't have the ability to see or feel things from another person's perspective. Never having experienced that kind of intense pain, nausea, weakness, and fear herself, Marci could not imagine what it felt like for her brother, and so she could not sympathize. She only knew how Brett's illness was affecting *her,* and that was what she reacted to:

> This was probably the most difficult time of my life. But it wasn't hard for me because I was grieving my brother. What was so hard was the loss of attention for such a long time.
>
> Brett had major mood alterations from his medicine. What had been a mischievous little boy who was fun to play with became a surly, rage-filled boy who started beating up his sister. This was also a mystery to me, but I blamed it on myself. I thought if I were nicer to him it would stop. As much as I tried, though, it seemed to get worse.
>
> What really got to me, then, was the fact that this person who was so mean to me was getting all the love and attention I was craving, while I was left wondering why I wasn't getting special meals, or having books read to me in the hospital, or having special quiet times on the couch with my own bell to ring in case I needed anything.
>
> I was just so sick of not being the "special sick boy." It seemed like he got *all* the special privileges. I wanted to be sick so bad.

How do families deal with jealousy when cancer moves into the house? The first step is simply to be aware that this is one of the side effects of being an invisible victim, and it is perfectly normal. If you are expecting this kind of effect, you'll feel more prepared for it when it happens.

It is also important to remind yourselves that younger children especially are just not able to step outside themselves and react to a situation selflessly. They do not have the emotional experience required to be truly sympathetic, so it is fruitless to hope for it. Do what you can to explain the changes that are going on in your family, but try not to tell your children how they should feel about the situation. Let them be angry or jealous or frustrated, and allow them to talk about those feelings if they need to. If you don't have the emotional strength to talk with them, try to find a friend or relative who can listen and respond sympathetically.

Outsiders, too, can learn to be more sensitive to the feelings of jealousy that commonly aggravate the cancer situation. Marci recalls how well-intentioned family friends only hurt her more.

There were very few people who were concerned with me, and I suppose they didn't think of me (since I was so young) as someone whose feelings they would have to consider.

Everywhere I went—church, school, the grocery store—there were hundreds of grown-ups who would recognize me, walk up to me, and the first words out of their mouths were, "How's Brett doing?" Most of them didn't even know my name.

They never asked me what my name was, didn't ask me how many letters I knew, or if I had gotten any new toys lately. I didn't matter to them except for what

I could tell them about Brett—which was a sore spot with me anyway.

I have said this earlier, but I want to repeat it: If you know someone who is suffering from cancer, be aware of the invisible victims too. Because it is terribly difficult for children to have to sacrifice some of the love and attention they depend on from their parents, it is common for them to be intensely jealous of the cancer patient. In spite of the genuine concern you feel for the patient, you may want to temper your curiosity when you're around his or her children or siblings. You might try asking about school, or sports, or pets, or books instead. If the children *do* want to talk about cancer or the patient, let them tell the story from their own perspective, expressing their feelings and revealing what's important to them personally.

> Does Jesus care when my heart is pained
> Too deeply for mirth and song,
> As the burdens press, and the cares distress,
> And the way grows weary and long?
>> O yes, he cares! I know he cares!
>> His heart is touched with my grief;
>> When the days are weary, the long nights
>>> dreary,
>> I know my Savior cares.
>>>> Frank E. Graeff

Jealousy may seem like an inappropriate response to cancer, but is it really all that long ago that you wished for a broken leg so you could have crutches? Or that you wanted your tonsils out so you could eat your fill of ice cream? Before becoming exasperated with how selfish your children may seem, try to see the situation from their point of view.

5

Facing Fear

No! This can't be happening to us, to me! There must be some mistake! This was Ellie's reaction when she learned that her husband, Howard, had cancer. She wanted to deny it, partly because she was deeply afraid of the profound changes that cancer would bring to her life.

Fear is common whenever humans are forced out of the familiar. And cancer in the family has a way of turning the familiar on its head. Ellie describes some of the feelings she experienced when cancer moved into her household:

For many days after my husband's cancer was diagnosed, I vacillated between denial and acceptance.
I struggled to come to grips with this big change in
my life.

Our family had just moved from Michigan to Illinois
five months earlier, and I didn't even know people
yet or have a support group to fall back on. I didn't
even know where the hospital was where his surgery
would take place. The fears kept welling up within
me about what I would do or where I would go if
Howie died. I didn't even have a home to call my own
because we lived in a church-owned parsonage. And
these fears were all the more intense because children were involved.

Whether a cancer patient lives or dies, the effect
of cancer on a family is life changing. Routines,
responsibilities, and relationships change. And
often there isn't time to make the adjustment gradually; the family is rudely shoved into unfamiliar
territory. Each day becomes an emotional chal-
lenge and a spiritual battle, and each person struggles in different ways. At the very least, the family's cancer experience is unsettling. More often it
is absolutely terrifying!

But Ellie found peace during her most fearful
times:

The prayer support of family, friends, and people
from many different churches became very evident.
The peace that surrounded us helped us move from
denying to accepting the reality of cancer. We asked
a lot of "whys" and felt that it was all right to ask, as

long as we did not rebelliously demand an explanation from God.

We cried a lot! We prayed a lot! And with each passing day, our faith was renewed, and we were strengthened.

Besides support from the Christian community, Ellie also found herself inspired by her husband's courage and positive attitude:

One day Howie looked me in the eye and said, "We will celebrate our twenty-fifth wedding anniversary." That was a turning point in my attitude. I could look at a future again. Now we give thanks that the Lord has blessed us, and we have just celebrated our thirty-fifth anniversary!

Fear is normal for any family dealing with cancer. In fact, underlying fear can be the root of many of the other stresses, conflicts, and negative emotional energy that seem to characterize the cancer experience and tear families apart. Recognizing the power of fear can be the first step in releasing your family from fear's grip. Admit your fears. Name them and face them. Talk about them with each other and with friends. Pray about them alone and together. As Ellie and Howard learned, "This can be a time in which a family learns to express their love and dependence on God."

And remember that we can be sure we are never left to face our fears alone. God's promise in Isaiah reads:

"Fear not, for I have redeemed you;
  I have summoned you by name;
    you are mine.
When you pass through the waters,
  I will be with you;
and when you pass through the rivers,
  they will not sweep over you.
When you walk through the fire,
  you will not be burned;
  the flames will not set you ablaze.
For I am the LORD, your God,
  the Holy One of Israel, your Savior . . ."
                          Isaiah 43:1–3

The psalmist offers us this simple testimony:

I sought the LORD, and he answered me;
  he delivered me from all my fears.
                          Psalm 34:4

6

Help from the Classroom

My husband and I have been blessed with good schools and professional, compassionate teachers for our children. The way they responded to our special situation made me aware of the important role a teacher has in a child's life. Here are some tips I would like to pass along to teachers whose students may be affected by cancer.

1. Make yourself knowledgeable about the situation. Know what type of cancer is being dealt with and what kinds of treatments are being prescribed. Try to get this information from the original source by keeping in touch often—don't depend on the grapevine or prayer chain.

2. *Talk with the child about the situation.* Take the time to ask what's going on at home and to listen to the child's perceptions of life with cancer. Be concerned with how the child is feeling and what he or she is thinking. When you notice deviations from "normal" behavior, handle it sensitively and recognize that this child is trying to cope with difficult and unfamiliar emotions.

3. *Let the child talk about the situation.* Of course, not all children will *want* to talk about how cancer is affecting their lives and their families, but some children may appreciate the opportunity. By letting a child address the class and answer questions, a teacher can replace an atmosphere of awkwardness and discomfort with an atmosphere of mutual openness and support.

4. *Express your support through cards and phone calls.* Teachers are extremely busy, but taking the time to make special contact with the family or an individual child is genuinely appreciated.

5. *If appropriate to your school situation, use the opportunity to teach your students about prayer.* Children need to learn early the purpose and power of prayer. Praying about cancer can teach children that answers do not always come quickly and that they are not always what we hoped for when they do come. During such a

confusing and painful time, a child may not *feel* God's presence or comfort. This may provide an opportunity to teach that our relationship with God does not make us immune from various kinds of suffering, and that our feelings do not determine whether or not God cares about us. Studying some of the psalms is a good way to open up discussion about God's faithfulness even when we feel abandoned.

> Answer me when I call to you,
>   O my righteous God.
> Give me relief from my distress;
>   be merciful to me and hear my prayer.
>
> Know that the LORD has set apart the godly for
>   himself;
>   the LORD will hear when I call to him.
> I will lie down and sleep in peace,
>   for you alone, O LORD,
>   make me dwell in safety.
>   Psalm 4:1, 3, 8
>
> I waited patiently for the LORD;
>   he turned to me and heard my cry.
> He lifted me out of the slimy pit,
>   out of the mud and mire;
> he set my feet on a rock
>   and gave me a firm place to stand.
> He put a new song in my mouth,
>   a hymn of praise to our God.
> Many will see and fear
>   and put their trust in the LORD. . . .

45

Many, O LORD my God,
  are the wonders you have done.
The things you planned for us
  no one can recount to you;
were I to speak and tell of them,
  they would be too many to declare. . . .
I desire to do your will, O my God;
  your law is within my heart. . . .
Do not withhold your mercy from me, O LORD;
  may your love and your truth always protect
    me.
For troubles without number surround me;
  my sins have overtaken me, and I cannot see.
They are more than the hairs of my head,
  and my heart fails within me. . . .
But may all who seek you
  rejoice and be glad in you;
may those who love your salvation always say,
  "The LORD be exalted!" . . .
You are my help and my deliverer;
  O my God, do not delay.
                    Psalm 40:1–3, 5, 8, 11–12, 16–17

6. Involve the class in the situation. You might
want to give the whole class an opportunity to
make and send cards or notes to a classmate's
family member. Not only is this an effective spirit-
lifter for the patient, it's also a way to give the child
some of the attention he or she may be craving.

I know that children in "cancer families" will
benefit from their teachers' skillful and sensitive
handling of their special situations, but I am also
sure that other children in the class will benefit

as well. By teaching compassion, prayer, and practical expressions of support, teachers can equip their students with skills they will need throughout their lives in dealing with their own trials as well as the trials of others.

7

Learning to Lean

One thing about life is this: It can be very humbling. It's natural to want to feel as though we have some measure of control—over our bodies, our families, our careers, whatever. But dealing with cancer is one way to be reminded that we are not in control. This lesson quickly becomes most obvious for the patient. As I wrote in my previous book:

> It was easy to feel like I was not in control of my life after cancer entered it. The cancer seemed to take

over everything. My time was no longer my own—
my schedule now revolved around treatments and
appointments. My thoughts weren't my own—the
cancer filled my mind despite my efforts to think
about anything else. My emotions were controlled by
both the cancer and whatever drugs were a part of
my treatment. Even my body wasn't my own—after
surgery and weight loss and nausea and the disease
itself, I didn't look much like the person I used to be.

But "control" is an issue that family members
and friends of a cancer patient also have to deal
with.

Kay is one woman who had to learn about surrender when her younger sister was diagnosed
with cancer in 1990. Kay was the oldest child in a
family that had experienced its share of heartache
and tragedy. A younger brother was retarded, and
Kay helped care for him. A second brother became a policeman and was killed in the line of
duty. Kay's father was plagued with frequent ill-
nesses and numerous surgeries. Her mother was
worn down by the many difficulties she had faced.
As the oldest child, Kay felt responsible for showing strength and leadership in helping to ease the
family's burdens.

So when her sister discovered she had cancer,
Kay's immediate reaction was to try to take control of the situation. "Being the oldest," she says,
"I honestly felt this was my job—to be there for
my sister, to save my mother, to support my

brother-in-law, to explain death and dying to my grown children—all as an example of being a great Christian."

Kay knew—had always known—that she needed to depend on God. But knowing that and living it are two different things. "I had put on a wonderful *fake* Christian face," she remembers. "I prayed the expected prayers. I referred to God's will and his presence in all circumstances. But still I thought, 'If I can't do what needs doing, then who will?'" Kay was not willing to "turn over the reins" to God. She had acknowledged God's will, but she hadn't surrendered herself to it.

Overwhelmed by the emotional and spiritual responsibilities she had put on herself, Kay finally—gradually—did reach a point of surrender. She explains:

> I can't name the time or the exact place, but slowly a new idea began to form in my mind: "If there is a God"—and I hoped there really was one—"and if I take the lost, overwhelmed child in me to the Father in him, and if I just tell him how mindful I am of my feelings and how selfish I feel, maybe he will work with me."
>
> He did! He told me every day, "I am here! I love your family *better* than you can! Let *me* be with them. I *know* where they hurt—you can only guess. Your sister is mine. She will come home to me. Don't ask why; it isn't for you to understand. I am the Father, and you are my child. You have been very grown up for a long time, and now I am telling you that *I* am the Father

and *you* are the child. Let me lead. Stop and listen. I have given you all that you need, and together you and I will take one day at a time."

Learning to surrender is a lifelong struggle that all Christians go through. But God demands it of us because he knows the blessings that come when we truly trust him—blessings like peace, reconciliation, healing. When I finally surrendered to God's will for my life and my cancer, I found a strength I couldn't have found within myself. I found a peace that was all-consuming and solidly powerful. And I found healing for my spirit as well as my body.

> What a fellowship, what a joy divine,
>   Leaning on the everlasting arms;
> What a blessedness, what a peace is mine,
>   Leaning on the everlasting arms.
>   Leaning, leaning, safe and secure from all
>   alarms;
>   Leaning, leaning, leaning on the everlasting
>   arms.
>
> Oh, how sweet to walk in this pilgrim way,
>   Leaning on the everlasting arms.
> Oh, how bright the path grows from day to day,
>   Leaning on the everlasting arms.
>   Leaning, leaning, safe and secure from all
>   alarms;
>   Leaning, leaning, leaning on the everlasting
>   arms.

What have I to dread, What have I to fear?
Leaning on the everlasting arms.
I have blessed peace with my Lord so near,
Leaning on the everlasting arms.
Leaning, leaning, safe and secure from all
alarms;
Leaning, leaning, leaning on the everlasting
arms.

Elisha A. Hoffman

Kay learned to surrender too. And she found a comfort she hadn't felt in a long time: "I may be the oldest in the family, but now I've learned I am not in charge of everybody's pain or joy. There is a child in me that needs the Father, and I am welcome to take all of me to him—especially the parts I am most ashamed of."

She also developed a deeper, richer relationship with her sister than she had ever had before: "God helped me make a best friend of myself for my sister. We finally said 'real' things to each other. She knew I cared even though I couldn't change anything." In fact, Kay's whole attitude toward the cancer was redeemed when she learned to surrender. She says today, "Without her cancer we may have lived to a very old age and never cared much about each other. For this I can be grateful for the cancer."

Of course, learning to lean is a process, not a one-time victory. The need for control is a natural human tendency, and surrender goes against who we are and everything we've learned. I still struggle to live the faith that I say I have, to feel confident in God's ability to run my life. But God always manages to remind me that he is running my life, whether I let him or not. Sometimes his reminders are dramatic, as I explained when I wrote about a spot that appeared on my sternum eight years after I had been declared cancer-free:

> This is the kind of uncertainty I live with every day now. It is a frustrating test of my willingness to totally surrender. Even when I think I'm cured, the threat of recurrence is there. My semiannual bone scan reminds me that, in a sense, I never leave the valley of the shadow of death. My life now is never my own; I can never regain the feeling of control that I had before I got cancer.
>
> Maybe that's good. None of us really control our own lives, though we like to think we do. And while it's frustrating for me to have to be continually reminded of my mortality, it's an important lesson to learn. God is in control.

I thank God for that!

8

Where Is God?

"Where is God?" you may ask yourself from the bottom of the pit you're in. "I hurt so bad, and there doesn't seem to be any comfort anywhere. Doesn't he hear me? Doesn't he care? Didn't he promise never to leave me?" You're angry. You're wounded. You feel betrayed.

Maybe you even doubt whether there is a God. Of course, you always knew there would be trials in your life—but this one feels so devastating! And all those promises and assurances you've read in

55

the Bible somehow sound hollow from where you're at now. You don't *feel* the peace that God promised. You haven't found the answers that he guaranteed. Now you're wondering, while the earth quakes under your spiritual feet, if your entire religious life has been nothing but a house of cards. *Where is God?*

Your doubts about God are real and not at all uncommon. Humans are sensory beings. We depend on what we can see and hear and touch to navigate our course in the world. As soon as something doesn't feel like we expect it to, we begin to doubt. Even so, God knows our doubts. And he accepts them. He is not shocked by the fierceness of your anger or the depth of your despair. In fact, he's had all those feelings himself. If you express your feelings to him honestly, he will listen without judging, and then he'll show you the way back to faith and strength. God understands.

In the midst of all your apprehensions, you can slowly learn to surrender to him. The paradox is, you can doubt him and trust him at the same time.

> I heard the voice of Jesus say,
>   "Come unto me and rest;
> Lay down, thou weary one, lay down
>   Thy head upon my breast."
> I came to Jesus as I was,
>   Weary and worn and sad;

Where Is God?

I found in him a resting place,
And he has made me glad.
Horatius Bonar

God hears your cries. He has always heard the cries of his children. And he has always reached out to save us.

If you are an innocent victim of this world's worst nightmares, at the very least you are probably questioning your relationship with God. You may feel that he doesn't understand you, or even that he's betrayed you or is not as real as you need him to be. But this God has suffered just as you have. He, too, was an innocent victim of abuse, anger, loneliness, and humiliation. He never deserved his pain.

You may be confident in God's life-changing power, or confused by his apparent silence. You may understand what he's up to, or you may not. Either way, he *is* the only answer to your pain. So let go of your expectations and turn to God with your anger and doubts. He alone is the source of healing, peace, and new life.

How long, O Lord? Will you forget me forever?
How long will you hide your face from me?
How long must I wrestle with my thoughts
and every day have sorrow in my heart?
How long will my enemy triumph over me?

Look on me and answer, O Lord my God.
Give light to my eyes, or I will sleep in death;

my enemy will say, "I have overcome him,"
   and my foes will rejoice when I fall.

But I trust in your unfailing love;
   my heart rejoices in your salvation.
I will sing to the LORD,
   for he has been good to me.

Psalm 13

9

Using Your Pain

An age-old question that has been debated and written about by scholars, philosophers, and theologians much wiser than I is "Why does God allow suffering?" There are, I think, a lot of answers to this question, a lot of good reasons for suffering. Some of them have been addressed in books like Philip Yancey's *Where Is God When It Hurts?* and James Dobson's *When Life Doesn't Make Sense.* But, of course, the answers we come up with are only educated guesses at best. Paul tells us in Romans 11, "Oh, the depth of the riches of the wisdom and knowledge of God! How unsearchable his judgments, and his paths beyond tracing out!" (v. 33).

When people start asking "Why?" the answers don't always come right away. The "good reasons" are not always obvious. But in my case, years after my diagnosis, I can see a purpose for my suffering: God allowed me to suffer so that I could minister to others who suffer. As Paul writes, "Praise be to the God . . . of all comfort, who comforts us in all our troubles, so that we can comfort those in any trouble with the comfort we ourselves have received from God. For just as the sufferings of Christ flow over into our lives, so also through Christ our comfort overflows" (2 Cor. 1:3–5). Can it be any clearer than that?

I have met hundreds of people since my own battle with cancer. I have counseled them on the phone, visited with them personally, sent cards and letters, made public speeches, given radio interviews, and written a book to share my experiences and feelings. People have told me that I have been a blessing to them in a very dark time of their lives. But I could not be this blessing if I hadn't been through the darkness myself. God is teaching me to use my pain to help heal others.

God began teaching the same thing to Les in 1993. Les, a pastor, remembers vividly the day he received the news that cancer had invaded his life:

My wife and I both walked silently out of the doctor's office to our car. We couldn't talk. We both hurt badly. I finally broke the silence by asking my wife how we should tell the children. It was then that my emotions got the best of me, and I broke down in tears.

My wife asked me to pull the car over and let her drive, but I rejected that offer. I had to show her I was fine, I was brave, I was still in control.

When we got home, I walked to the office thinking I could put some finishing touches on the sermons I had to preach in a few days. But I couldn't put my mind to work. Instead I picked up the phone and called a good friend. I told him as best I could what the doctor had told us. Less than an hour later, he and his family were at our house. We couldn't talk much, and there were long periods of silence, but it was very evident that they shared the grief that was in our hearts. It meant a lot to us. It was good to feel the support of a loving family in that particular hour of need.

This man's ministry was never quite the same after that. By personally facing and enduring faith-shaking pain and fear, Pastor Les became a "wounded healer," a phrase first used by Henri Nouwen in his book by that name. Today Pastor Les says:

All pastors should be wounded healers, even though many have not had the same experience I had with cancer. Pastors must be people who have felt the wounds of loneliness, alienation, separation, isolation, rejection, failure, and pain. Pastors must be aware that God uses these wounds to make us wounded healers.

The primary ministry of the pastor is not to take away the pain. Pain is good because it points us to the pain reliever, Jesus Christ. The task of the pastor is to prevent people from suffering for the wrong reasons, and to remind them that all of us are mortal and broken and that there is a liberation only Christ can give. In this liberation there is hope, and hope is what suffering people need more than anything else.

Often, a wounded healer is just one who is there, creating an atmosphere and an opportunity to allow the emotions of the patient to flow, and giving him the assurance that no matter how dark the future may be, there is One who goes with us.

Of course, people like Pastor Les and me can encourage other cancer patients because we have experienced the cancer battle. But another ministry that is often overlooked is the ministry to family members and other invisible victims of the cancer experience.

Marci (you may remember her from chapter 4) was able to use her pain to comfort another family when the father in that family developed leukemia. She was only fifteen years old when this man, her cello instructor, was diagnosed. Her youth and her own experience with her brother's leukemia uniquely equipped her to meet this family's needs. She wrote at the time:

My teacher's wife told me that he honestly thought he was going to die in the near future and that he was not sleeping at night or anything—he had changed because of this sickness. I was aghast. She herself was not far from being completely unnerved. I told her then of my brother's experience with this sickness and tried to relay my confidence in her husband's recovery.

It seemed to help a bit, but the most significant thing about this encounter was that this was when I committed myself to helping these people through this. No matter what, I was going to see this thing to the end. This couple needed someone to count on, and—God help me—I was going to be the one. Since then I have tried to help them in every way I could. Sometimes it meant baby-sitting for free, sometimes skipping lessons because he was in the hospital, and sometimes just "being there."

I think my knowledge of the disease and its effects on people helped them because they had no idea if his particular case was abnormal or not. And it gave them some "inside information," for instance, that a particular drug reaction would be loss of appetite, and that his shakes were only a reaction to his medication.

Perhaps most significantly, Marci could minister to the children of this family in a way that no one else could:

I tried my hardest to help his children because I know firsthand what they were going through. I could see Nathanial [the son] begin using enormous amounts of physical aggression just to get some plain affection. I could also see that his acting up did not accomplish this, because it annoyed his frazzled parents. I am teaching him that fighting does not work, and that if he wants a hug, just ask for it. It has been working too. The last time I was over there, which was last Friday, he sat on the couch and snuggled with his sister and me without fighting or trying to hurt her. The best part about it was that he really enjoyed just being close, which rarely happens in families that are involved with serious diseases.

Maya [the daughter] had begun withdrawing because she also wanted some attention and love. Tears were in her eyes almost constantly, and whining soon became her normal tone of voice. I had a hard time seeing that happen because this girl reminded me so much of myself when I was a child. We, Maya and I, understand each other now. I make her laugh, and I listen to what she says and let her sit on my lap, and she doesn't whine anymore. In fact, she has become amazingly strong emotionally. I am proud of them both.

Beautiful things can happen when we use our pain to comfort others. Terri, another invisible victim, remembers, "We noticed that the most supportive people were the ones who had already experienced trials themselves." The fact is, pain exists. There's no escaping it. Every human will be introduced to some form of suffering at some point in his or her life. Whether or not that's fair or necessary is irrelevant; it's reality. Our questions and complaints won't change that reality.

What we *can* change are the results of that reality. If you, like me, are a cancer patient, you can reach out to other cancer patients in a way that no one else can. You can meet needs and express feelings that those outside of the cancer experience may not even be aware of. You've been given a unique gift—the gift of empathy.

Or if you, like Marci, have been indirectly attacked by cancer, you too are in a strategic position. You've been given eyes to recognize the invisible victims of cancer, and you can draw from your own pain to comfort others who suffer in a similar way.

You probably won't be able to use your pain right away. It's difficult to be a healer when you haven't healed yet yourself. But once you are able, take any opportunity you can to comfort another sufferer. I know of no better way to turn Satan's destroying darts into a healing balm.

Blood Brother
The Bible paints a picture
of an involved
and compassionate God.

From the very beginning,
when he stooped down
on hands and knees
in the dust
and stuff of earth
to form
fashion
with his own hands
man,
he has known us absolutely.

His commitment is so intense
so actual
that he willingly forced himself

into a human body,
a specific lifespan,
and lived like us,
felt all the things we feel.

His own pains
were not somehow
easier
because he was God.
He was not stoic and passionless.
No, he thundered and wept.
He laughed and feared.
And,
at the end,
drenched with sweat,
he trembled and begged,
"Please don't make me die!"
He screamed in agony
and cried out tearfully,
"Oh God! Where are you?"

This God knows pain.

Your pains
now
are just as real to him.

He suffers *with* you
at every twist of life.

The pains
and frustrations
and heartbreaks you go through
exist
not as proof that he doesn't care,
but as a part of life

Using Your Pain

so significant
that removing them
would make you *less*.

Rather than effortlessly banishing pain,
God has chosen to share it
intimately
with you.

See the scars on his hands?

Melanie Jongsma
As Real As You

10

Let's Talk about It

In October of 1985, two years after my diagnosis, my husband wrote me a letter in which he opened his heart and worked through some of his feelings. I have treasured it ever since. Following are excerpts from Jim's letter:

Dear Bea,

We have a special relationship. We have established a family that is unique and special. We have nurtured and trained our children. We have a lot to look forward to in the area of family—graduation, Jon's marriage, college for Jayne and all the good experiences that will bring, grandchildren, Jon's business and his success, Jackie's high school years, then her college years and all her activities. These are times when we as husband and wife have to grow closer together. In a sense we have to grow away from being parents of younger children, but now parents of adult children. I say this knowing that we will always be nurturing, caring parents to our children regardless of their age.

We have each other to love and cherish. We should continue to be best friends, to share our mutual concerns, to grow together as a Christian couple. I need to be sensitive to your needs and feelings, give encouragement when you feel down, help you when you feel overwhelmed—like I did when you were going through the treatments. That really was a special time.

I remember you lying in the hospital in Decatur, anticipating the surgery, or, going back even farther, getting the report from Dr. Helms and driving back to the hospital. Dr. Helms had said the tumor was cancerous and you would need more surgery. I had WMBI [a Christian music station] on the car radio at the time, and I don't remember the song, but I had to turn it off because it made me cry.

That whole period of time was a very dark time of our life. Until then we had never had to deal with cancer. In fact, the word *oncology* was new to our vocabulary. Cancer was something other people got. Now we had to face it. To me, the word *cancer* was synonymous with the terminality of life.

I questioned how our family would deal with this intrusion in our life. There was a lot of uncertainty connected with it. I don't think that I really could possibly feel how you felt because it was your life which was being threatened.

The surgeries were uncertain. Lymph node involvement made the outcome uncertain. Even this summer you were frightened when you had a broken rib because of weakness in that area. I can't really feel how you felt, but I can sympathize with you.

I am really glad that you are doing well. You're a good wife and mother to our children. I'm happy with our children and a lot of the credit has to go to you.

God in His wisdom has brought us together, and therefore we should not resist, but press on to reach the goal of more perfect communication and openness.

Love,
Jim

I cannot overemphasize the role my husband played in my recovery. As I recuperated from that first surgery in the Decatur hospital, Jim and I shared a special closeness and began forging a bond that would withstand all the fear and frustration and weariness that we didn't even know were yet to come. We spent many hours alone together, trying to come to grips with our new life and our changing relationship.

I applaud my husband for his honesty and openness, for setting a high standard for our relationship and helping us both to meet it. One reason our marriage is strong today is that Jim has the courage to talk about his feelings—the positive and the negative. We share our dreams and discouragements. We bear our burdens together.

And now it is important for me to remember to support Jim. He, like our children, is an invisible victim and probably has some residual emotional issues to deal with. The invasion that cancer has been in our marriage continues today; in fact, to a great extent it defines who we are and how we relate to each other.

But Jim reminds me to keep striving to meet that standard he set all those years ago in his letter to me, the standard of "more perfect communication and openness." We will not let emotional issues go underground, we will not allow resentments to build, we will not let cancer—or anything else!—come between us. Our response to conflict is: "Let's talk about it. Let's pray about it."

Thank you, Lord, for blessing me with such a wonderful life partner!

It is important that cancer patients express thanks and appreciation to the invisible victims for the support given, and also be sensitive to their fears and anxieties.

I urge family members to be open about their thoughts and feelings, as painful as this sometimes is to do. There is much to be gained in support, affection, and mutual understanding with openness. If it is difficult for you to talk about your feelings, ask for the Lord's help and he will direct you and give you the right words to say. You'll be happy you made the effort to communicate, and you may even make some precious memories in the process.

11

Stress Relievers

Undeniably, terminal illness will bring a great deal of stress to your family. Not only is there a great volume and variety of emotion being spent, but the physical demands of battling cancer impact the entire family as well as the patient. Here are some things I learned about handling and relieving stress:

1. Prayer is powerful. Focus on the Lord, who heals all our diseases and redeems our lives from the pit. Focus on his Holy Spirit, the Comforter and Encourager. Acknowledge your doubts, fears, and anger, and surrender them all to him. Find a quiet place and a quiet time to be alone with God.

Try not to let anything rob you of this time—remember, even Jesus needed prayer!

2. God's Word is relevant. I found an amazing wealth of verses that seemed to be describing exactly my feelings and circumstances. Often, my children or family friends would jot down some Scripture on a card or in a note and share it with me. Many of these I have committed to memory, and I am still blessed by their messages today.

3. Advice and support are important. Don't be afraid to confide your feelings to friends you can trust. At the very least, you may find it comforting to know that what you're experiencing is a normal reaction to a difficult situation. If you or members of your family are dealing with difficult emotions, like depression or denial, or if you simply need support, you might want to take advantage of the services of a Christian counselor or pastor who will help you put your feelings in perspective.

4. Attitude makes a difference. Try to be positive. This doesn't mean you should deny the seriousness of the situation or ignore the negative feelings you may be having. It is only a reminder to be aware of God's blessings and his answers to prayer. Look for something to praise God for—you might even want to make this exercise part of your family devotions or bedtime tuck-in ritual.

5. The physical affects the emotional. Remember to pace yourself. It is not healthy to operate in high gear at all times. If you let your body get run down, your emotions will soon follow. Try to get enough sleep and maintain a nutritious diet. In the same way, it is not healthy to "idle" all the time either. Spending most of the day in bed, even spending most of the day indoors, can intensify your feelings of depression and helplessness. Get up on time, keep a schedule, do something physical, go somewhere different. Exercise is a great stress reliever.

6. *Families are made up of individuals.* Even though you are all going through the same trial, each of you will react in different ways. Don't expect your entire family to be "on the same page" at the same time. Allow each person the freedom to feel his or her own emotions and to express them appropriately.

7. *Arguments drain emotional resources.* This may seem obvious, but when a family is going through emotional upheaval, arguments can seem impossible to avoid. Still, avoiding them is often the healthiest choice. Defend the values you know are important, but don't waste time and energy arguing over trivial issues. Do what you can to keep your relationships mutually supportive.

8. *In giving, we often receive.* You might feel absolutely unable to even *notice* someone else's pain, much less offer healing. Then again, you might be surprised. By reaching out to someone else in need, you may find refreshing relief from your own concerns.

If your family is feeling the pain of dealing with cancer, encourage every member to look at this list of stress relievers and adopt some of these suggestions. Don't let stress rob you of the strength you will need to find emotional and physical healing.

12

Journaling

*N*ot *everyone* likes to write, and when you're going through depression, disease, grief, and stress in general, it may seem like a lot of extra work to keep a journal of the experience. But I have found journaling to be a great stress reliever, as well as a written record of God's faithfulness. For those reasons I recommend journaling to anyone dealing with cancer—patients as well as their families.

Cheryl kept a journal while her father was suffering from cancer. Of course, the experience was painful and heart wrenching, but today she is glad she has a record of it. She says:

> The whole experience was so painful that I blocked out a lot of it. That's one of the reasons for writing

these memories on paper—in hopes to forget for "the now." But yet they're not gone forever, because I know I have them journaled down. Reading them now, I recognize some of the smaller details that help me to recapture the memories more clearly. I had forgotten in the two years that have passed. I'm glad I journaled my experiences and some of my thoughts.

Journaling doesn't have to be a rigid discipline. You may feel like writing every day, or you may only write every now and then. Whatever you do, don't worry about spelling, grammar, punctuation, or any of the other things you've been trained since grade school to be concerned about. Your journal is for *you,* no one else.

"But what do I write?" This is the most common question I hear from people who have never been in the habit of journaling. Since getting started is the hardest part, I'll list some ideas that may help. Once you're off and running, though, you'll probably never again feel intimidated by a blank sheet of paper!

> *Write a letter to God.* Tell him how you are feeling—and be honest! Ask for his help and strength.
>
> *Write a letter to an unknown person.* Tell him or her about your appearance, your background, your activities and interests, your opinions and feelings, your home life, your family and other significant people, your fears and dreams. This

kind of letter is fun to go back to every few months because it's a way of tracking whether your perception of yourself has changed.

Write the phrase "I am . . ." ten times. Then go back and finish each sentence.

Draw a pie chart of your day, showing all the activities you engage in and how much of your time they absorb—eating, sleeping, writing letters, going to work or school, and so on.

Write a letter to yourself.

Write a letter to your family doctor. Describe how you feel about the treatments, his or her manner, and the prognosis. Remember, you don't have to send this letter, so be as unrestrained as you want!

Draw a line down the middle of the page. On one side list things you like about yourself. On the other side list things you don't like. Praise God for the things you like and ask for his help in changing the things you don't.

Make a list of things you're angry about. Rate them on a scale of 1 (mildly upset) to 10 (screamingly furious!). Then pray that God will work with you to replace your anger with peace and forgiveness. Of course, coming to a point where you are spiritually healed enough to *feel* this peace may take a long time, but don't give up.

Write a letter to someone who has had a major influence on your life.

Write "I wish . . ." and "I need . . ." ten times and finish each sentence.

Ask yourself some profound questions. For example: Why am I here? What is most important to me? What beliefs am I willing to stand up for? What sacrifices am I willing to make for those beliefs? What makes me happy? What is love? What is death? What do I believe about heaven?

Write down some of your favorite Scripture verses, poems, or song lyrics.

A journal is a great place to share your highs and lows with yourself and with God. It is a safe place to vent some scary feelings, a record of how you handle good days and bad days. And it can be a chart of your own spiritual progress and God's answers to heartfelt prayers. Try it!

13

When Death Is at the Door

It's hard to admit and difficult to talk about, but death is a real possibility for every cancer patient. I believe in the power of positive thinking, and I believe that God answers prayer, and I believe in miracles. But I also know that not all cancer patients get better. Sometimes they die.

One milestone in the battle against cancer is knowing when to concede defeat. That may sound like fatalism or heresy, but it is reality. In fact, it is reality whether or not you have cancer. Death awaits each of us; denying that truth only

limits the time and energy we have to prepare ourselves for it.

Conceding defeat may be especially difficult
for the family of a cancer patient. Loved ones
often consider it their responsibility to encourage, cheer, and support the patient, whatever the
circumstances may be. So when the patient be-
gins talking about death, the family's typical first
reaction is to try to talk him or her out of it. At
times this tactic may be appropriate because an
occasional reference to death may simply be a
symptom of weariness or depression, and the family members should do what they can to coun-
teract that. Other times, though, impending death
is not just a possibility but a reality that needs to
be accepted by patient and family alike. If you
find yourself in this situation, you might find the
following suggestions helpful:

1. Don't be afraid to talk about death. Refusing
to bring the subject out in the open only makes
it more terrifying. And as Christians we have a
great deal to say about death that is *not* frighten-
ing, sad, or hopeless.

One night shortly after my initial diagnosis and
my return from the hospital, I was unable to sleep.
I walked through the house, peering out the win-
dows and into the empty night. My son, Jon—in
high school at the time—came downstairs and
saw me. He told me he couldn't sleep either. "I
feel like someone died," he said. I told him I felt

the same way. We had no idea what the future would hold for our family, but we felt the ominous closeness of death.

I'm glad Jon was able to share those feelings with me that night. In response I turned on a Christian radio station whose *Songs in the Night* program featured gentle arrangements of comforting psalms and hymns. Jon slept on a pillow in front of the stereo for the rest of the night. He had faced his grief and found a measure of peace in doing so.

2. *Don't cling to false hope, and don't encourage others to do so.* It is not uncommon for cancer patients to have an inner sense of their condition and prospects. They may know, if they are honest with themselves, when things are not going well. A healing family will respect such feelings and give patients the freedom to express them openly.

3. *Know when it's time to let go.* One "advantage" of a terminal illness is that it gives a person time to say good-bye. If you, as a family member, are refusing to accept the oncoming death of your loved one, you are only making it more difficult for him or her to face the end. Sandi remembers the conflicting reactions of her parents to her father's diagnosis:

In my mind, from day one I totally accepted death. But not Mom or even Dad at first. She tried to get him to eat and exercise to get his strength and weight back. For me it was real frustrating to see the battle between them. Finally, toward the end, I had a confrontation with Mom. I asked her why she was pushing and forcing him to eat and exercise. She said it was good for him and the doctor said he needed to gain weight. At that point I said, "Dad is not going to get better. Just let him do whatever he wants." All this was taking place in front of Dad. He agreed. It was time for them to let go and let the cancer take its course.

This may be the most difficult part of the struggle, but it is so important. Patient and family have to know when to let go. Talk about how you will miss each other, about how afraid you are, about any regrets you have. If you can't talk or cry in front of each other, write a note, or just spend time being together. By accepting the inevitability of death together, you can make your last shared moments precious, instead of wasting them wrapped in denial.

> I stand at the edge of the Jordan River,
> watching its cold, dark waves deliver
> someone I love to the other shore—
> a parting I thought I'd prepared myself for.
>
> The haze and the grays of the cool dawn hide
> what I want to see of the other side—
> an easy arrival, a welcome embrace,
> an unhurried walk to a beautiful place.

But whether or not I can see it, I'm sure.
In spite of my questions, my faith is secure.
Whether or not I see it, I know.
But still I resist when it's time to let go.

M.J.

4. Take care of business. Death's approach makes us keenly aware of things we have left undone or unsaid, believing we would get around to them sooner or later. But cancer's physical effects on a person may make it difficult for the victim to take care of this unfinished business without help. If you are close to someone who is dying, look for an opportunity to volunteer your assistance. You may be able to help write or deliver a letter, set up a meeting between friends, make financial or legal arrangements, organize a vacation—something to help fulfill an unrealized dream or take care of an unfinished matter. If you are the cancer patient yourself, don't be embarrassed to ask for a friend's help if you need it. Settling all your practical *and* emotional accounts will give you peace of mind and may leave your loved ones something comforting to remember you by.

5. Don't be afraid to be physical. There's no denying that thinking about death makes us uncomfortable. And it is not uncommon for family members to deal with the threat of loss by avoiding the situation and even the very person whose death seems imminent. Working long hours, surrounding ourselves with busyness, or retreating emotionally and physically are ways of avoiding the idea of death. Of course, ultimately no one can avoid death, and the excuses we make only rob us of precious moments with a person we love.

Try to overcome your apprehension by maintaining physical contact with the cancer patient. Give hugs and handshakes just as frequently as you ever did. You may find that addressing the situation in a direct, physical way will help you overcome your fears and ease the tension for everyone concerned.

6. Pray for strength. Death is our last and greatest enemy, and facing it is an emotionally, physically, and spiritually draining ordeal. Whether you are the patient or a family member, don't forget to refresh your spirit through prayer, and enlist others to pray for you as well.

It is difficult to discuss the positive side of death without sounding trite, but this eternal hope for us is so very real. Death has been swallowed up in victory! We *will* meet our loved ones again on the other side. Knowing this may not minimize the pain you are going through now, when death is knocking at the door, but at some point you may be able to return with confidence to the comfort and hope of Jesus' promises:

"I tell you the truth, whoever hears my word and believes him who sent me has eternal life and will not be condemned; he has crossed over from death to life."

John 5:24

14

Facing the Future

Too often it's true that bad things happen to good people. While God gives each of us a certain measure of control over our lives, the consequences we endure don't always match the choices we make. As your parents may have told you, "Life is not always fair."

Why is that? Because our world is torn between opposing forces. While God is the ultimate ruler, there is an enemy who desperately struggles to wrestle our lives out of God's hands and ruin his plans for us, his children. That's why our plans sometimes fail and our dreams may turn to dust. That's why life isn't "fair" and bad things can happen to good people.

But God *is* in control. It may seem sometimes that he's no longer interested in us, that he's left the world to spin itself wearily into hopeless ashes, while hordes of fearless demons dance in victory. But things are not always what they seem. God is continually at work to bind those singing demons and restore this fallen world to its potential glory. In spite of how your life looks right now, God is in control, and with him you *can* face the future with hope.

The Bible tells the story of a man named Job, whom God put through a series of fiery trials for reasons Job couldn't understand. Job spent years wondering, "But *why*, Lord?" In the end he learned that he didn't have to know the answers. He only had to believe that God is in control. Having passed the test, Job found the peace he needed.

The same will happen for us as we choose to expand our trust in God beyond our human perception. The apostle Paul reminds us, "No eye has seen, no ear has heard, no mind has conceived what God has prepared for those who love him" (1 Cor. 2:9).

Are *you* afraid of the future? Do you wonder what life holds for you and your loved ones? Do you worry about what lies ahead? Facing the unknown is often disturbing and sometimes terrifying. But if your heart belongs to God, you can see beyond your situation today. You can know for sure what your future holds:

> **Q.** What is your only comfort in life and in death?
> **A.** That I am not my own, but belong—body and soul, in life and in death—to my faithful Savior Jesus Christ.
>
> He has fully paid for all my sins with his precious blood, and has set me free from the tyranny of the devil. He also watches over me in such a way that not a hair can fall from my head without the will of my Father in heaven: in fact, all things must work together for my salvation.
>
> Because I belong to him, Christ, by his Holy Spirit, assures me of eternal life and makes me whole-heartedly willing and ready from now on to live for him.
>
> *Heidelberg Catechism*

Trust Jesus. He suffered untold agonies, died to pay for our mistakes and to redeem for us the life we hold so dear. He took the sting out of death and the fear out of the future. Let him fill you with his peace and comfort you with his promises. Besides giving you confidence in your eternal destiny, trusting all your *tomorrows* to him can give you the strength you need to face anything *today*.

> Great is Thy faithfulness, O God my Father! . . .
> Pardon for sin and a peace that endureth,
> Thine own dear presence to cheer and to guide,

Cancer Lives at Our House

Strength for today and bright hope for tomorrow,
Blessings all mine, with ten thousand beside! . . .
   Great is Thy faithfulness!
   Morning by morning new mercies I see;
   All I have needed Thy hand hath provided,
   Great is Thy faithfulness, Lord, unto me!

Thomas O. Chisholm

Epilogue

We, as a family, are thankful for God's guidance and protective care over us. We have found that it is possible to emerge from a devastating life situation as whole persons, reconstructed and refined by God through our trials.

Our lives have been touched and permanently changed by the cancer experience. But it has been a joy to watch God take a devastating, life-threatening experience and work it out for something positive and good.

Our family has been built up in our love for God and each other, and we all look forward to carrying out the rest of his plan for our lives.

Appendix

Helpful Resources

Publications

Collins, Gary. *Spotlight on Stress*. Santa Ana, Calif.: Vision House, 1983.

Hoek, Beatrice Hofman, and Melanie Jongsma. *Surrender or Fight? One Woman's Victory over Cancer.* Grand Rapids: Baker, 1995.

Hoeksema, Herman. *Meditations: God Is Our Refuge and Strength.* Grand Rapids, 1946. (Copies obtained by writing South Holland Protestant Reformed Church, 16511 South Park Avenue, South Holland, IL 60473.)

Jongsma, Melanie. *Stress: Letting Go and Letting God.* South Holland, Ill.: The Bible League, 1993.

———. *Talking with God.* South Holland, Ill.: The Bible League, 1992.

Komp, Diane M. *A Child Shall Lead Them: Lessons in Hope from Children with Cancer.* Grand Rapids: Zondervan, 1993.

———. *A Window to Heaven: When Children See Life in Death.* Grand Rapids: Zondervan, 1993.

McNamara, Jill Westberg. *My Mom Is Dying: A Child's Diary.* Minneapolis: Augsburg Fortress, 1994.

Meier, Paul D. *Meditating for Success.* Grand Rapids: Baker, 1978.

Minirth, Frank B., and Paul D. Meier. *Happiness Is a Choice: A Manual on the Symptoms, Causes, and Cures of Depression.* Grand Rapids: Baker, 1978.

Reisser, Paul. *Energy Drainers, Energy Gainers.* Grand Rapids: Zondervan, 1990.

Schaeffer, Edith. *Affliction.* Old Tappan, N.J.: Fleming H. Revell, 1978.

Siegel, Bernie S. *Love, Medicine, and Miracles.* New York: Harper & Row, 1990.

Simonton, Stephanie Matthews. *The Healing Family.* Los Angeles: Bantam Books, 1984.

Smedes, Lewis. *How Can It Be All Right When Everything Is All Wrong?* New York: Harper & Row, 1982.

Vanderwell, Howard D. *Proven Promises.* Hudsonville, Mich.: 1990.

Vogel, Linda Jane. *Helping a Child Understand Death.* Philadelphia: Fortress Press, 1975.

Support Groups and Hot Lines

The American Cancer Society. 1-800-ACS-2345 (or write to the ACS at 777 Third Avenue, New York, NY 10017 [local units are listed in your telephone directory])

The National Cancer Institute. 1-800-4-CANCER

Y-ME. 1-800-221-2141

❈ ❈ ❈

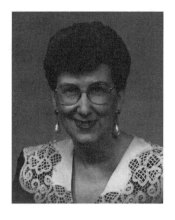

Beatrice Hofman Hoek is an energetic teacher, homemaker, mother, and grandmother who does not intend to let cancer dominate her lifestyle. **Melanie Jongsma** is an editor at the Bible League, has written several books, and assisted Bea in writing her story. They make their homes in Chicago's south suburbs.